Available in Paperback and Kindle Version
Amazon.com

DEDICATION

TO MY HERO, MY SON SAM MCNEES

A million thanks to Dr. Monisha Crisell at TriValley Urology, Dr. Christopher Kane and Dr. Michael Albo at University of San Diego Medical Center, the staff at Moores Cancer Center and UCSD Thorton Hospital. Also, thanks to Kevin the CT Scan guy!

Beautiful Cancer

How to Embrace One of Life's Greatest Challenges

Defining a Beautiful Approach to a Cancer Diagnosis

AUTHOR JAMI BUCHANAN MCNEES

I see trees of green

Red Roses too

I see them bloom

For me and you

And I think to myself

What a wonderful world

Louis Armstrong

Contents

BEAUTIFUL CANCER

WHERE TO BEGIN AND HOW TO SPEED READ THIS BOOK

When I received my diagnosis, I was in panic mode. I was constantly doing Google searches in hopes of finding something that would tell me what to do, how to prepare or what I could expect. I wanted answers and I wanted them fast, simple and bullet pointed. So, to honor you and the possibility that you too are in panic mode and have stumbled onto this writing while anxiously Google searching for answers to handling Cancer, I have designed the following information in a simple bullet pointed format for your convenience. Each section will begin with a Concept, followed by the backstory on how the Concept was formed, then a repeat/reminder of the Concept. **IF YOU WANT TO SPEED READ THROUGH THE ENTIRE BOOK IN 10 MINUTES AND JUST GET THE GENERAL CONCEPTS, THEN SPEED THROUGH THE CONTENT BY READING ONLY THE BOLDED UPPERCASE TEXT.**

I AM THE MOST FORTUNATE WOMAN IN THE WORLD AND OTHER AWESOME ATTITUDES

WHEN DIAGNOSED WITH CANCER, YOU CAN MAKE A CHOICE. FOCUS ON THE DARKNESS OF THE SITUATION OR FOCUS ON THE LIGHT SIDE, THE BRIGHTER SIDE. I SAY, "WALK TOWARDS THE LIGHT, BABY!" FIND THE POSITIVE IN EACH SITUATION. THERE IS ALWAYS SOMETHING, NO MATTER HOW LITTLE, THAT IS POSITIVE OR FORTUNATE ABOUT EVERY CIRCUMSTANCE. LOOK FOR THAT LITTLE RAY OF LIGHT. THEN CHASE IT AND I PROMISE YOU WILL FIND MORE LIGHT!

Cancer Journeys should not be compared, one to another, even though some are clearly more difficult and take a life far too early. But as cancer experiences go, I consider mine to have been quite easy (and yes, that is probably a big dose of Survivor's guilt talking). It wasn't easy because it was physically painless. It was easy because I embraced the experience as part of life. Some say that attitude is everything. Others say Cancer doesn't give a crap about your attitude. For several years, I have had a personal mantra I mentally repeat on sleepless nights, or while on the massage table or when I wake up from a Sunday afternoon nap. I AM THE MOST FORTUNATE WOMAN IN THE WORLD. Even after my diagnosis, I still believed I was the most fortunate woman in the world. I had supportive friends and family, I had Health Insurance, I had access to great doctors, I had money in the bank and I was self-employed working from home. Talk about fortunate!

Part of the surgical procedure to remove Bladder Cancer and reconstruct my body was a radical Hysterectomy which included removing most of my vagina. "Go ahead and take all the lady parts!" I told my Doctor. "I haven't used them in years." Having the vagina removed might be a crisis for a married woman with a virile husband. But not me! I'd already been happily single for 13 years and had just recently concluded that I truly never wanted to remarry. The Lady Pleasure Palace was closed for business! The Honey Pot was history! Now, thanks to the Hysterectomy, I'll never have to worry about Cervical Cancer or Pap smears ever again! I am the most fortunate woman in the world!

I can't be sure if it was the euphoric effect of pain killers or deep sincere gratitude that caused me to feel like I was the most fortunate woman in the world immediately after my surgery. It was probably both. I would nap every day in my easy chair covered with the handknitted afghan Jackie made me when I was first diagnosed. I felt covered in love. My little dog snuggled in my lap and Downton Abbey videos were cued up on the DVR. Never mind that my abdomen was covered in medical tape and wads of gauze or that I had tubes dangling from multiple places in my abdomen leading to bags of bodily fluids lying on the floor next to me. I still felt like the most fortunate woman in the world. I was recovering from Cancer surgery in my happy place surrounded by the love-saturated walls of my cozy little home. Behind my easy chair, resting on the mantel, were photos of my tiny family over the years and vintage glamorous photos of my mom looking over me. It was Springtime. Birds chirped, breezes blew through new leaves, and my wind chimes pinged and ponged their calming peaceful music. I believed without a doubt, I was the most fortunate woman in the world.

Maybe they're right. Attitude is everything.

I AM THE MOST FORTUNATE WOMAN IN THE WORLD

WHEN DIAGNOSED WITH CANCER, YOU CAN MAKE A CHOICE. FOCUS ON THE DARKNESS OF THE SITUATION OR FOCUS ON THE LIGHT SIDE, THE BRIGHTER SIDE. I SAY, "WALK TOWARDS THE LIGHT!" FIND THE POSITIVE IN EACH SITUATION. THERE IS ALWAYS SOMETHING, NO MATTER HOW LITTLE, THAT IS POSITIVE OR FORTUNATE ABOUT EVERY CIRCUMSTANCE. LOOK FOR THAT LITTLE RAY OF LIGHT. THEN CHASE IT AND I PROMISE YOU WILL FIND MORE LIGHT!

CONCEPT ONE

CHANGE THE LABEL OF CANCER. MY CANCER EXPERIENCE WAS BEAUTIFUL

Pema Chodron teaches about labeling the events in our lives.

Recall the feeling you have when you are lying in bed snuggled under your covers and you hear it raining outside. Mmmmm, you think to yourself, "How wonderful." But what if you wake up one morning and you hear it raining outside and it's your wedding day? You think to yourself, "This is awful!" It's the same rain, but because you have labeled it either good or bad, you have determined in advance the role, the effect and the impact it will have in your life.

I knew I had Cancer even before I received the diagnosis. I decided to label it as one of the greatest life adventures I could be gifted.

I don't like suspense. Maybe you don't either. So, let's start with the end of the story. I had invasive Bladder Cancer. I had a radical 9-hour surgery to remove the bladder, 20 lymph nodes, my ovaries, my uterus, my cervix and most of my vagina. Then the surgeon repurposed healthy intestine to make a new internal reservoir to replace the bladder. I have a stoma (hole) in my abdomen that provides access to the new reservoir using an 18-inch catheter multiple times a day to remove urine from my body. And I lived happily ever after. The end. Yay me!

So why am I writing? Because in comparison to the fear, dread and darkness associated with Cancer, my Cancer experience was amazing, beautiful, wonderful and fulfilling. How is it that my experience could be so radically different from the stories one usually hears about Cancer? For a while, I thought it was because my Cancer was no big deal and not as bad as everyone else's Cancer. I opted out of chemo and was spared the pain of chemotherapy and its horrible side effects. But then I remind myself that I will pee through a tube for the rest of my life and that the lady pleasure palace (vagina) is closed for business permanently. And I think, huh, when you put it that way, it sounds bad...very bad. So, yes, my Cancer was a big deal with long term life-altering consequence. Then why do I feel like it was so awesome? How is it that my experience was so Beautiful?

(Before I continue, I'd like to insert a caveat right here!!! Every cancer journey is different. My experience and my suggestions are in no way intended to reduce or minimize the pain and desperation others have experienced. Each of us does the best with what we have, where we are in the time and space we given. I honor every Cancer patient)

Perspective is everything. If you believe an experience is beautiful, then you will have a beautiful experience. If you believe an experience is tragic then you will have a tragic experience. You will always find exactly what you are looking for.

We approach each new life experience based on the history of all the events leading to this moment and how we perceive the world. Sparing you the details, I will simply say we all have peaks and valleys in our life history. I had my share of both ups and downs. But perception is everything and I am a lover of self-help books, and motivational podcasts. So, at the time of my diagnosis, I was more than just a "glass half full" kind of gal. I was "my cup runneth over" optimistic "grab the golden ring" Pollyanna kind of gal. My cancer journey started with a wonderful level of optimism already installed. As a result, my cancer experience was awesome, wonderful and beautiful. But if you have been diagnosed with Cancer and can only see it from a place of doom and gloom, keep reading. Hopefully you will find ways to see it from a new perspective.

CHANGE THE LABEL OF CANCER. MY CANCER EXPERIENCE WAS BEAUTIFUL

Take a moment...write your thoughts or pause for reflection.

Think about how you have labeled your experience until now. How do you wish to label your Cancer Journey in the future?

CONCEPT TWO

GO STRAIGHT TO ACCEPTANCE

YOU HAVE TWO OPTIONS FOR DEALING WITH CANCER. YOU CAN CHOOSE TO ACCEPT YOUR DIAGNOSIS WITH COURAGE AND DETERMINATION AND FIND WAYS TO THRIVE OR YOU CAN RESIST YOUR DIAGNOSIS AND LIVE IN DENIAL AND ANGER. ONE OF THOSE OPTIONS IS FAR MORE EFFECTIVE THAN THE OTHER.

Receiving a Cancer diagnosis thrusts you straight into the 5 stages of grief, sorrow and loss. Those stages are denial, anger, bargaining, depression and finally acceptance. Each stage can take hours, days or weeks.

DENIAL – "The Doctor read the test wrong. This must be a mistake. I demand a second and third opinion."

ANGER (and blaming) – "I'm a good person. How could this possibly happen to me? I don't deserve this! This is Bull S&%$. The Doctor is an idiot. He has no idea what he's doing. It's his fault. He should have caught this earlier."

BARGAINING – "I swear, if I survive this, I'm going to be a vegan, sugar-free, alcohol-free organic Yogi Master and read my Bible every day starting right now. Are you listening God? Please do a miracle and take this away from me. I promise I'll be a better person."

DEPRESSION – "I give up. I feel hopeless."

ACCEPTANCE – "I have Cancer. I didn't anticipate this, but I am willing to adjust my life to increase my odds of survival and thrive through this experience."

What if you skipped over the first four stages and started with the fifth stage? What if you started with ACCEPTANCE? It worked for me.

The condensed version of my story: My one and only symptom was bright pink pee. Pink pee was enough for me to make an appointment to see my Family Practitioner who referred me to a Urologist.

There was a week lag time before my visit to the Urologist. This provided me an entire week to consult Dr. Google. Entering *pink pee* in the Google search bar kept giving me info on Bladder Cancer, its symptoms, its treatment, its prognosis. I mentally filed these Google searches under "Oh Shit" and "Oh my God" and "Holy Crap".

My Urologist appointment was uneventful but didn't sound very promising. She wanted to do a CT Scan and a cystoscopy in which the doctor can view the interior of the bladder from a tiny camera. There was another week lag time between the appointment and the tests in which I did more Googling and Cancer kept appearing in my search results.

As I drove myself to the appointment for the CT Scan and the up close and personal camera angle of my bladder, my thoughts drifted. I don't know how to explain it, but I calmly became very aware that I had Cancer and the tests were going to confirm what my body was telling me and my heart already knew. I knew enough about Cancer (thanks Dr. Google) to realize that almost 40% of people will be diagnosed with some form of Cancer in their lifetime. That's a huge number. Based on that statistic, instead of thinking "Why me" I thought "Why not me". Who am I to be spared the odds of almost 1 out of 2 people? Alone in my car, armed with a considerable amount of online research about Bladder Cancer symptoms, and with only my Creator listening, I said out loud "I have Cancer. Now what am I going to do about it?"

The imaginary voices of Pema Chodron (a Buddhist teacher), Sheryl Sandberg COO of Facebook, and Oprah answered back to my "now what" question. I very calmly said out loud, to myself and my Creator, "Okay. Let's do this, Lord. I accept I have Cancer. I'm going to embrace it, lean in to it, learn amazing life lessons and have an awesome over the top incredible life adventure named Cancer that not everyone gets the privilege to experience. And then I'm going to survive and live happily ever after. So, bring it on. Let's do this."

My doctor confirmed I had bladder cancer.

I didn't feel sad. I didn't feel scared. I ACCEPTED it. My body and my heart already knew I would be a survivor. I was determined.

YOU HAVE TWO OPTIONS FOR DEALING WITH CANCER. YOU CAN CHOOSE TO ACCEPT YOUR DIAGNOSIS WITH COURAGE AND DETERMINATION OR YOU CAN RESIST YOUR DIAGNOSIS AND LIVE IN DENIAL AND ANGER. ONE OF THOSE OPTIONS IS FAR MORE EFFECTIVE THAN THE OTHER.

Take a moment...write your thoughts or pause for reflection.

Where are you in your Acceptance of your diagnosis? Denial? Anger? Bargaining? Acceptance? Where would you like to be? What would it take to get you there?

♥

CONCEPT THREE

GIVE CANCER THE SPACE AND HONOR IT DESERVES. FIVE MINUTES A DAY IS A GOOD PLACE TO START.

CANCER DESERVES TO BE HONORED AND RESPECTED. SETTING ASIDE TIME EACH MORNING TO ARTICULATE YOUR FEARS AND VERBALIZE POSSIBLE SOLUTIONS MAY HELP THE FEARS STOP SWIMMING AROUND IN YOUR HEAD.

There were a few other tests and bone scans that needed to be done to confirm my cancer was limited to the bladder before I could be scheduled for outpatient surgery to remove the tumor. But I was confident that I was going to be Bladder Cancer's winning poster child for what I called "One and Done". I'd have outpatient surgery and this would all be history. After only two weeks of my diagnosis, I was already shopping on Amazon for Cancer Survivor T-shirts.

I've heard of people who make Cancer their identity and carry it like a load they must suffer. I'm not criticizing. We all process our situations differently. But, I wasn't interested in making the burden of Cancer any portion of my identity. I wanted to be strong and independent. So, I kept my diagnosis on the down low. I told my family and my closest friends. But, I didn't want to be viewed as a Cancer patient or victim by my community.

Truthfully, I didn't have time for Cancer when I was first diagnosed. I had more exciting things going on in my life. I was in my busiest selling season of the year and the phone was ringing off the hook. I might be able to squeeze Cancer into my calendar later, but not at that moment. I figured Cancer didn't pop up overnight, so there was no need to rush to fix it immediately. Besides all that, in the bigger scheme of things, this was my life journey of many years, both past and future, and Cancer was simply visiting my body for a short-term ride along. I didn't see any reason to let the temporary passenger in my body dominate my life. Cancer's days were numbered. But it was Cancer, and you really can't ignore it.

Cancer, once diagnosed, won't allow you to ignore it. Even with my accepting lean in attitude, random fears would surface. "What if I have to have chemo and lose my hair? What if the final diagnosis is late stage Cancer and I need to wear a bag on my body filled with urine all the time? What if I lose my hair? (Yes, I know I already said, "what if I lose my hair", but it popped up all the time.) What if chemo makes me throw up a lot and frequently? I hate throwing up. What if I don't survive? What if I die?" It's hard to fully concentrate on anything when Cancer keeps demanding your attention and won't shut up.

I thought it would be helpful to process these fears in a productive manner rather than denying and stuffing them down. So, I decided that I would fully and intentionally focus on Cancer... but only for five minutes a day.

Each morning, after my coffee and before I started my work day, I would sit in an antique rocking chair that no one ever sits in and give Cancer the time, space, honor, attention and respect it deserves. I would mentally focus on the area of my body where Cancer was residing and would have a very serious audible conversation in my most sincere tone of voice. The conversation usually went something like this..." *Good morning Cancer. How are you this morning? I hope you are comfortable in there. It's rather warm and cozy isn't it. I'm glad you're here. I really am. I feel privileged. I thank you in advance for the wonderful things you will bring to my life. I'm sure you have some great lessons planned for me. I'm excited to learn and I hope to get the lessons right the first time. Please let me know if there is anything you need from me. I'd like to make your short journey with me as pleasant as possible for both of us. I've decided not to worry about chemo. I'll deal with it when it comes if it comes. But not now. I've already started a Pinterest Board of great wigs just in case. I'm going to buy an extremely expensive wig if I lose my hair. So, I don't need to worry about losing my hair. Check that fear off my list. As for the throwing up thing... I absolutely refuse to throw up. I've never smoked pot before, but I hear it helps with side effects of chemo. In the event of chemo induced nausea, I'm willing to light up a big fat joint if it will keep me from throwing up. If I don't survive this and I die...well, we all die sometime, don't we? But I really hope I don't die bald. It was nice visiting with you Cancer. I must go now. Your five minutes are up for today. I have a lot of important things to accomplish that don't include you. But I'll see you again tomorrow morning for five minutes. Cancer, you have a wonderful day. I know I will."*

Setting aside time each morning to articulate your fears and verbalize solutions may help the fears to stop swimming around in your head. Journaling might work better for you to organize your thoughts. But my thoughts were coming at me at the speed of a microwave oven and writing was too slow of a process for me. Whether you journal or talk to Cancer, the important concept here is to set aside intentional time to focus on Cancer.

A few times a day, Cancer would interrupt my thoughts and concentration and whisper in my ear "Holy crap Lady, you have Cancer!" I would take a deep breath and mentally respond as if Cancer was in the room with me, "Yes, I know. I'll focus on you again tomorrow for five minutes. But that's all you get."

I have a book club of business women who I love and adore. I walked into one of our meetings late and took a seat and listened while Tina was describing, in intricate detail, her current troubles related to her heart condition and the procedure that would hopefully resolve the issue. It was a very long explanation. When she was done, my friend Kelley looked over at me and said, "So Jami, update us on your health." I paused, smiled and said, "I can't update you now, I only give Cancer five minutes a day and it already had its time this morning." They all stared back at me waiting for more. There was silence in the room until Jeannette burst out a laugh. Tina looked at me and said, "I love it! I'm sick of talking about my heart. From now on it only gets five minutes a day." And then we talked about the book we read instead of talking about Cancer. I liked it better that way.

Five minutes a day, that's all I was willing to give Cancer.

GIVE CANCER THE SPACE AND HONOR IT DESERVES. FIVE MINUTES A DAY IS A GOOD PLACE TO START.

CANCER DESERVES TO BE HONORED AND RESPECTED. SETTING ASIDE TIME EACH MORNING TO ARTICULATE YOUR FEARS AND VERBALIZE POSSIBLE SOLUTIONS MAY HELP THE FEARS STOP SWIMMING AROUND IN YOUR HEAD.

Take a moment...write your thoughts or pause for reflection.

Create a routine to set aside quiet time each day to focus on your diagnosis either by journaling or talking to yourself. What is the best time of day for you to do this? Articulate your fears then create possible solutions? What advice or comforting words would you want to hear from a wise person who has already walked this path?

CONCEPT FOUR

FIND A TRAILBLAZER

FIND SOMEONE TO REFERENCE WHO HAS SURVIVED CANCER AND THRIVED. THINK OF THEM AS YOUR TRAILBLAZER AND FOLLOW IN THEIR FOOTSTEPS. IT CAN BE SOMEONE YOU KNOW OR A CELEBRITY WHO HAS A GREAT SURVIVOR STORY.

In the corporate world, it is highly recommended to seek a mentor. Find someone who has already achieved the goal to which you aspire. Watch them, shadow them, mimic them and learn from them. This will sky rocket your success. The same is true with Cancer. Find survivors that are thriving and mimic them.

Long before I was diagnosed, as I drove to work each morning, I would often see Marcy, a 20 something woman in my neighborhood walking her dogs. Marcy was bald from chemo but so strikingly beautiful I couldn't help but pause and stare. I was incredibly impressed by Marcy. She looked stunning, invincible and powerful. Years later, when I was diagnosed, I thought to myself, "I want to do Cancer like Marcy. I want to be as beautiful and as invincible as Marcy." Was it that Marcy was young and hip and could pull off bald like a runway model? Or was it her inner peace, living in the present and her Phuck Cancer strength that exuded from her every pore? Or was it her confident courageous determined defiant walk in the new morning sunshine that made her so beautiful? Maybe it was all the above. If I had to have Cancer, I wanted to be like Marcy.

I'm a Health Insurance Broker. Many of my every day conversations are with clients with histories of Cancer. One of them is Jen. She is a breast Cancer survivor. I met with Jen at her kitchen table to sign Medicare Supplement paperwork. She was a vibrant single woman, Realtor and dog breeder. Her house is as beautiful as a model home. Pictures of her adult children, dog portraits and breeder awards lined the walls. The space was filled with life and joy. When I was diagnosed, I thought to myself, "After this is over, I want to live a full wonderful life like Jen."

Alice is one of my clients with Cancer whom I have yet to meet face to face. Two years ago, before my diagnosis, her husband called me. In a calm, steady, low, quiet voice James said, "My wife has just been diagnosed with Breast Cancer. She needs surgery as soon as possible. I need to get her the best health insurance available." Alice's husband and I spoke many times a day that first week. I researched which Health Insurance companies contracted with the list of doctors James provided. I emailed him the results asap. He'd email me late in the evening with the names of more doctors, surgeons, specialists and hospitals. I'd do the research immediately and respond back again as soon as possible. He calmly asked questions about the impact of pre-existing conditions, health insurance coverage, reconstructive surgery costs, chemo costs and physical therapy. At the end of the week, James calmly selected the Insurance Company and policy that would be the best fit for his wife. I processed the application and Alice got the insurance she needed. But the experience of working with James touched me. I was moved by this man's calm Rock of Gibraltar strength in the face of crisis and possible unspeakable loss. He never expressed anger, frustration or fear. He was simply cool, calm and aware of what he needed to do. When I was diagnosed two years later, I thought to myself, I want to be strong, cool and calm like James.

I am grateful for my trailblazers who were shining examples creating powerful illustrations of how I would do Cancer. Before my surgery, I bought long flowing feminine skirts in anticipation of comfortably covering up the tubes and catheters that would help me heal. I felt lovely in spite of all the gauze, tape and tubes. I would be beautiful like Marcy. I put my house in order before I went into the hospital. It was lovely like Jen's. While recovering, I often woke up from my noon naps, sitting in my easy chair feeling fortunate, even blissful, to be healing in my beautiful little happy place. I kept calm through most of the experience and kept my focus on healing. I was strong like James. Thanks to my trailblazers, I knew how to do Cancer.

*names have been changed to protect privacy

FIND SOMEONE TO REFERENCE WHO HAS SURVIVED CANCER AND THRIVED. THINK OF THEM AS YOUR TRAILBLAZER AND FOLLOW IN THEIR FOOTSTEPS. IT CAN BE SOMEONE YOU KNOW OR A CELEBRITY WHO HAS A GREAT SURVIVOR STORY.

Take a moment...write your thoughts or pause for reflection.

Who do you know who has had Cancer that you might learn from or who might offer you inspiration? It could be a person you are acquainted with or a celebrity that is a Cancer Survivor? What is it about this person that you would like to imitate on your Journey?

♥

CONCEPT FIVE

NURTURE YOURSELF...RETREATING MAKES GOOD SENSE

SELF-NURTURING IS GOOD FOR THE SOUL EVEN WHEN YOU DON'T HAVE CANCER. BUT IT IS ESPECIALLY BENEFICIAL WHEN YOU HAVE BEEN DIAGNOSED. ALLOW YOURSELF PLENTY OF TIME TO HONOR YOUR EMOTIONS.

I'm part of a very large community of business networkers and close friends. During the holidays, there is a mixer or celebration two or three times a week. I loved getting out of the office and mixing it up socially with these great people. Normally, I thrive off their energy.

But it became very awkward, at these networking events, when people would approach me, give a little business appropriate hug, then ask the typical greeting, "Hi, how are you? What's new?" Awkward silence on my part followed. I mean really? What was I supposed to say? Responding with my typical reply of "I'm great! How are you?" seemed incredibly disingenuous. I felt awkward. Do I tell them? Do keep it a secret? What should I say? Informing them of my diagnosis while celebrating the holidays didn't feel like a good fit. I didn't want to talk about Cancer and I didn't want to dampen the enthusiasm of the unwitting acquaintance who was just trying to make conversation. Mixers and holiday celebrations just weren't the time and place to tell people I had Cancer.

Having Cancer, even when you have a positive attitude about the freaking awesome experience you're in the process of navigating, is a big load to carry. It's not appropriate for casual conversation. So, I opted out of mixers and holiday parties to avoid the discomfort of carrying on surface social banter and the awkward energy needed to keep my secret. I chose, instead, to stay home and be gentle with myself and enjoy some personal nurturing. Lavender scented baths, Haggen-Dazs ice cream and Downton Abby reruns were my self-indulgences of choice.

Self-nurturing is good for the soul even when you don't have Cancer. But it is especially beneficial when you have been diagnosed.

So, I decided to relax more. Life was on a new trajectory and no longer normal. Uncharted territory is awkward and exhausting. It was time to put my needs first. Retreating to my Happy Place, was ideal for this Introvert. But if you are an Extravert, alone time is the last thing you need. If you need nurturing and people, make an appointment at a Day Spa and invite friends to be with you. Go to the busiest mall filled with people and window shop. There are no right or wrong options here. The important thing is that you find a way to nurture your soul.

NURTURE YOURSELF...RETREATING MAKES GOOD SENSE.

SELF-NURTURING IS GOOD FOR THE SOUL EVEN WHEN YOU DON'T HAVE CANCER. BUT IT IS ESPECIALLY BENEFICIAL WHEN YOU HAVE BEEN DIAGNOSED. ALLOW YOURSELF PLENTY OF TIME TO HONOR YOUR EMOTIONS.

Take a moment...write your thoughts or pause for reflection.

What are your favorite ways to nurture yourself? Set aside time to find ways to indulge in some of your favorite foods or activities.

CONCEPT SIX

CRYING AND CUSSING ARE THERAPEUTIC. EMOTIONAL PREPAREDNESS IS ESSENTIAL.

THERE WILL BE TIMES AFTER A CANCER DIAGNOSIS, WHEN YOU NEED TO SLOW THE DOCTORS DOWN SO THAT YOU CAN EMOTIONALLY CATCH UP TO THE NEXT STAGE IN THE PROCESS. THIS IS YOUR JOURNEY. NOT THEIRS. IT'S OKAY FOR YOU TO DICTATE THE TERMS AND TIMING OF THE JOURNEY.

CUSSING AND CRYING ARE GREAT EMOTIONAL THERAPY WHEN YOU RECEIVE SAD NEWS WHILE ON YOUR CANCER JOURNEY. BUT AFTER YOU'VE CRIED AND RUN OUT OF F-BOMBS, CATCH YOUR BREATH, ATTEMPT TO SEE THE BIGGER PICTURE AND COUNT YOUR GOOD FORTUNE. GOOD FORTUNE IS STILL ALL AROUND YOU.

My fears and tears surfaced the morning of the outpatient surgery. I was nervous. I was scared. The process was supposed to be simple. Take out the tumor and send me home a couple of hours later pumped up on pain killers. Extra strength Tylenol would be all I would need to relieve the discomfort the following day. Then, check in with the Urologist a week later to get the pathology results. I was confident that I was going to be Bladder Cancer's winning poster child for what I called "One and Done". I'd have the outpatient surgery and this would all be history.

Things don't always go as planned with Cancer. The tumor wasn't easily removed. I was completely unprepared for the catheter attached to a urine collection bag I had to wear for more than a week. I confess my deep intense hatred for catheters right now! I was miserable all day every day.

Finally, my friend Jackie drove me to my post-surgery follow up appointment and I told her I'd call her when I was ready to be picked up. I practically kissed the nurse who removed the catheter. Did I mention catheters are hell on earth? Once removed, I just wanted to bask in the freedom and relief of no more catheter. My doctor came in, opened her computer, reviewed the pathology report and very calmly told me my Cancer was angry, aggressive and invasive. Invasive meant that Cancer had moved past the wall of my bladder and they had not been able to remove the tentacles of the tumor. There was still more cancer. Then she delivered the news that I would need a lengthy surgery to remove the entire bladder and do a radical hysterectomy. The recovery time could take 6-8 weeks. Then she looked me straight in the eyes, made sure I was paying attention and sympathetically said, "We're going to have to remove most of your vagina." Time stopped. My hearing became muffled as if I was under water. They are going to remove half of my WHAT? She suggested we call the surgeon right away and set an appointment for a consultation.

Whoa! Just whoa! I wasn't emotionally prepared for any of this. I told her I needed time to process what she had just told me but I promised I would call the surgeon in the next couple of days.

There will be times after a Cancer diagnosis when you need to slow the doctors down so that you can emotionally catch up to the next stage in the process. This is your journey. Not theirs. It's okay for you to dictate the terms and timing of the journey.

I walked out of the office in shock and with eyes as big as saucers. Jackie was waiting for me curbside. I climbed in her car and warned her she was about to see something rarely seen by any other human being. I was going to Ugly Cry. "Jackie, the Cancer isn't gone. It's invasive. They have to remove everything, even my vagina." I put my face in my hands and sobbed loudly. Jackie is a world class crier so she wept with me. What a great friend she is. When the tears slowed we started to cuss like drunken sailors. "Bleep it tee Bleep bleepin Cancer! This is so Bleeped up! Bleep this Bleepin Bleep"! Slight pause to wipe a tear. "Bleepin bleep bleep bleep! What the Bleep! Holy bleepin bleep!"

Even with all the cussing and crying, before we had even left the parking lot, I realized how fortunate I was. I didn't need to worry about the expense of more surgery. My Health Insurance would cover 100%. How fortunate. I was a Health

Insurance Agent and already knew that my insurance allowed me to see the best doctors and hospitals. How fortunate. I was self-employed and worked from home so I could easily accommodate a lengthy recovery period. How fortunate. I had already completed menopause, lost my sex drive and had decided I didn't want to date anymore! Heck! They could take my entire Vagina! I didn't need it any more. No vagina? No problem! How fortunate. The tears stopped. We cussed some more as we drove to my house. Jackie offered to stay but I let her know I would be okay. I called my sister and delivered my bad news. Then drove to the local nail salon and had a pedicure. I needed nurturing. A good long foot soak and new polish seemed like a great option. Except for some more bleeping texts back and forth with Jackie, I stayed quiet and low key the rest of the day. I needed to give my emotions time to catch up to this new direction of my Cancer Journey.

CRYING AND CUSSING ARE THERAPEUTIC. EMOTIONAL PREPAREDNESS IS ESSENTIAL.

THERE WILL BE TIMES AFTER A CANCER DIAGNOSIS WHEN YOU NEED TO SLOW THE DOCTORS DOWN SO THAT YOU CAN EMOTIONALLY CATCH UP TO THE NEXT STAGE IN THE PROCESS. THIS IS YOUR JOURNEY. NOT THEIRS. IT'S OKAY FOR YOU TO DICTATE THE TERMS AND TIMING OF THE JOURNEY.

CUSSING AND CRYING ARE GREAT EMOTIONAL THERAPY WHEN YOU RECEIVE SAD NEWS WHILE ON YOUR CANCER JOURNEY. BUT AFTER YOU'VE CRIED AND RUN OUT OF F-BOMBS, CATCH YOUR BREATH, ATTEMPT TO SEE THE BIGGER PICTURE AND COUNT YOUR GOOD FORTUNE. GOOD FORTUNE IS STILL ALL AROUND YOU.

Take a moment...write your thoughts or pause for reflection.

How are you processing this very emotional time in your life? Find a way to express your emotions either by talking to a friend or in a support group.   How are you emotionally preparing for the next step of your Cancer Journey?

♥

CONCEPT SEVEN

WORDS HAVE POWER

FRAME YOUR CANCER WITH WORDS AND IMAGES THAT CONJURE UP FEELINGS OF INSPIRATION, PEACE AND JOY INSTEAD OF FEAR AND DREAD.

WORDS HAVE GREAT POWER WHEN YOU ARE DIAGNOSED WITH CANCER. CHOOSE YOUR WORDS WISELY SO THAT YOU MIGHT EXPERIENCE CANCER IN A SPACE FILLED WITH JOY, PEACE AND GOOD FORTUNE.

In the beginning, I thought my Cancer experience would process fast like a Cancer Walk for Life 5K Event. Commit to the Walk, ask for support from close friends and family, show up, walk 5K, get the T-shirt, go home declaring mission accomplished. Early in my diagnosis, only my closest friends and family knew I had Cancer. I wasn't afraid to reach out to those I was closest to. I felt their love and support immensely. That was enough. But when the diagnosis changed to Invasive, I felt like I was preparing for a Marathon instead of a short 5K race. I had my little support system in place, but the extended version of my journey would have bearing on how I functioned in the large community in which I socialized. What was I supposed to do with this new diagnosis? Should I continue to only share the info with my closest friends and family? Kim, a very valued friend of mine, is the Executive Director of a Breast Cancer Resource Center. We sat across from each other at a business luncheon. During our conversation, she mentioned that the women who struggle with PTSD after cancer are the ones who kept it secret out of shame or not wanting to burden others.

I felt very uncomfortable sharing this very personal experience with mere acquaintances. But, I also realized that sharing my burden would lighten my load and reduce the stress of secret keeping. I had no desire to add PTSD to my list of symptoms now or later. So, I decided to share my circumstance with my very large community of friends and acquaintances through Facebook. But it needed to be in my "language" using words that were true for me.

(Facebook post March 5, 2016) Words have power so I choose to frame my experience in words that resonate with me. When my doctor told me I had Bladder Cancer (November 2015) I chose not to battle it or struggle with it. Instead, I chose to honor it, value it, appreciate the lessons it would bring and embrace the hell out of the experience. January 2016 my Doctor described my Cancer as angry and aggressive. Those words just don't work for me. So, I choose to refer to my Cancer as super friendly, over achieving, shows a lot of initiative and strives for total success. I can respect that description. The next stop in my

adventure (late March) is Radical Surgery at UCSD Medical Center. Instead of Radical Surgery let's refer to it as the Ultimate Repurposing Project using healthy body parts to make a new bladder. How freaking cool is that!? I'm totally going to be Bionic! I sincerely find this totally and utterly fascinating.

Best part of this experience has been discovering that my son, Sam McNees is a tower of strength and compassion. Best discovery   ever!

So, what can you do for me? I'm glad you asked. Send me good vibrations, rub a rabbit's foot, pet a Unicorn (Tara, you can help with this), kiss an Irish woman (Jackie Steed can help with this part), pray to the Almighty and do a good deed in my name to add to my Good Karma account. Please, someone tell Tom Hanks that I will live for another 30 years just in case he ever becomes single again.

> *#EmbracingCancer*
> *#AdventureOfALifetime*
> *#EverythingIsALesson*
> *#ThankGodForHealthInsurance*
> *#SoonToBeBionic*
> *#JamiNewAndImproved*
> *#HellOfAWayToLose5Pounds*

My home was already filled with graphics printed with fancy fonts of positive messages about life. A large wooden graphic of Louis Armstrong's Wonderful World lyrics dominates the wall you see as soon as you enter my house, "*I see trees of green, red roses too, I see them bloom for me and you, and I think to myself, what a wonderful world.*" God, I love that song. In my living room above the TV screen hangs a wooden plaque with the line from a famous Christmas movie. The plaque reads "It's A Wonderful Life." I keep this plaque up all year round.

When my mind would start spinning with fear and worry, I would recite chants and mantras in my head such as, "I am made to live a long and healthy life" or "My body is a temple of peace and healing" or "I am the most fortunate woman in the world".

I have used self-hypnosis (also known as Neuro Linguistic Programming) in the past to change unproductive negative messages stuck in my subconscious. This consists of listening to a new positive message over and over and adopting new thought patterns. I was hopeful that I could find a pre-recorded positive uplifting cancer NLP message to keep my spirits up. But I was unsuccessful. The program I downloaded freaked me out! The disturbing words "fear and anxiety" appeared early in the recording. Instead of the recording bringing peace and calm, it triggered fear and anxiety. I never listened to the recording again. No negative language allowed!

WORDS HAVE POWER

FRAME YOUR CANCER WITH WORDS AND IMAGES THAT CONJURE UP FEELINGS OF INSPIRATION, PEACE AND JOY INSTEAD OF FEAR AND DREAD.

WORDS HAVE GREAT POWER WHEN YOU ARE DIAGNOSED WITH CANCER. CHOOSE YOUR WORDS WISELY SO THAT YOU MIGHT EXPERIENCE CANCER IN A SPACE FILLED WITH JOY, PEACE AND GOOD FORTUNE.

Take a moment...write your thoughts or pause for reflection.

Make a list of positive words and phrases you would like to use more often and a second list of words you'd like to eliminate. Print the positive phrases on brightly colored paper in big bold fonts and tape them where you will see them most often.

CONCEPT EIGHT

BE CAREFUL WHAT YOU PRAY FOR

WHILE YOU ARE ON YOUR CANCER JOURNEY, PRAY THAT YOU WILL BENEFIT FROM THE EXPERIENCE. PRAY THAT OTHERS AROUND YOU, WHO ARE ON A JOURNEY PARALLEL TO YOURS, WILL BENEFIT TOO. PRAY FOR WISDOM, STRENGTH, PATIENCE, LOVE, PEACE, UNDERSTANDING AND ENLIGHTENMENT.

PRAYER? BEFORE YOU START PRAYING FOR ME, WAIT JUST A DAMN MINUTE!

I believe in the power of prayer, but not like you might expect from a woman who grew up in a conservative evangelical church. I believe there is power in any conscious thought, wish or prayer we send out into the Universe or to our Creator. I believe that when people pray as a congregation, or gather together as a group with a common goal or purpose, or say the Pledge of Allegiance or stand and sing the Star-Spangled Banner, something powerful in this world shifts and moves. So, you must be very careful what you pray for. Especially when you are praying for another person.

I saw my Cancer diagnosis as an amazing life experience that would bring me many lessons that could transform me into a better human being. I choose to accept it and not try to pray it away. Yes, Cancer would be hard, but what great adventure isn't hard? There are no easy lessons. I chose to accept my diagnosis and let it change me. So, if any one was praying for a miracle to cure my Cancer, pray it away or relieve me from this challenge, I wanted to tell them to STOP IT! STOP IT RIGHT NOW!

Life is filled with ups and downs, highs and lows, peaks and valleys, laughter and weeping, love and hate, health and sickness. These are all part of the ride and adventure of the gift of life we've been given by our Creator. Trying to pray away the hard parts of life doesn't make sense to me...and I suspect, doesn't make sense to our Creator. It's all part of the process and experience we call life. We have each been given an amazing gift of Life. Every bit of it is wonderful and painful and messy and should be experience with our whole heart. My Cancer experience was an amazing experience, a wild ride, a thrilling adventure...and I was all in!

Our struggles in life occur when we attach labels to life experiences as either good or bad. We expect that we should only experience good in life and we try so hard to avoid the bad. But what if they are one and the same? I love the fable of The Farmer's Son.

The Farmer's Son

One day in late summer, an old farmer was working in his field with his old sick horse. The farmer felt compassion for the horse and desired to lift its burden. So, he left his horse loose to go the mountains and live out the rest of its life.

Soon after, neighbors from the nearby village visited, offering their condolences and said, "What a shame. Now your only horse is gone. How unfortunate you are! You must be very sad. How will you live, work the land, and prosper?" The farmer replied: "Who knows? We shall see".

Two days later the old horse came back now rejuvenated after meandering in the mountainsides while eating the wild grasses. He came back with twelve new younger and healthy horses which followed the old horse into the corral.

Word got out in the village of the old farmer's good fortune and it wasn't long before people stopped by to congratulate the farmer on his good luck. "How fortunate you are!" they exclaimed. You must be very happy!" Again, the farmer softly said, "Who knows? We shall see."

At daybreak on the next morning, the farmer's only son set off to attempt to train the new wild horses, but the farmer's son was thrown to the ground and broke his leg. One by one villagers arrived during the day to bemoan the farmer's latest misfortune. "Oh, what a tragedy! Your son won't be able to help you farm with a broken leg. You'll have to do all the work yourself, how will you survive? You must be very sad", they said. Calmly going about his usual business, the farmer answered, "Who knows? We shall see."

Several days later a war broke out. The Emperor's men arrived in the village demanding that young men come with them to be conscripted into the Emperor's army. As it happened the farmer's son was deemed unfit because of his broken leg. "What very good fortune you have!!" the villagers exclaimed as their own young sons were marched away. "You must be very happy." "Who knows? We shall see!", replied the old farmer as he headed off to work his field alone.

As time went on the broken leg healed but the son was left with a slight limp. Again, the neighbors came to pay their condolences. "Oh, what bad luck. Too bad for you"! But the old farmer simply replied; "Who knows? We shall see."

As it turned out the other young village boys had died in the war and the old farmer and his son were the only able-bodied men capable of working the village lands. The old farmer became wealthy and was very generous to the villagers. They said: "Oh how fortunate we are, you must be very happy", to which the old farmer replied, "Who knows? We shall see!"

I discovered that mine wasn't the only journey of my Cancer diagnosis. My friends and family were on a discovery journey of their own. They were becoming painfully aware that if it could happen to me, it could happen to them. My son's journey was the most frightening. His life was impacted more than anyone else. He suffered much more fear than I did. He was afraid my life would end. It was important for me to support him spiritually. So how does an all knowing, all powerful, all present loving God fit into Cancer? The answer depends on your faith and how you were taught to see God. Do you see Him as judgmental and punitive? Then you'll see your Cancer as punishment. Do you see Him as a loving compassionate Creator? Then you'll feel His warmth, compassion and presence with you on this journey. I knew that my Cancer diagnosis was an opportunity to experience a deeper level of life and feel my Creator's constant presence.

While you are on your Cancer journey, pray that you will benefit from the experience. Pray that others around you who are on a journey parallel to yours will benefit too. But do not try to pray away the amazing life changing opportunity and adventure of Cancer. Pray instead for wisdom, strength, patience, love, peace, understanding and enlightenment.

BE CAREFUL WHAT YOU PRAY FOR

WHILE YOU ARE ON YOUR CANCER JOURNEY, PRAY THAT YOU WILL BENEFIT FROM THE EXPERIENCE. PRAY THAT OTHERS AROUND YOU WHO ARE ON A JOURNEY PARALLEL TO YOURS WILL BENEFIT TOO. PRAY FOR WISDOM, STRENGTH, PATIENCE, LOVE, PEACE, UNDERSTANDING AND ENLIGHTENMENT.

Take a moment...write your thoughts or pause for reflection.

What have your prayers been like so far? Are you begging God to take this away? Take a moment now to pray for peace, wisdom, strength, love, patience, understanding and enlightenment.

CONCEPT NINE

BECOME YOUR OWN ADVOCATE

BE YOUR OWN ADVOCATE. THIS IS YOUR JOURNEY. DO YOUR OWN RESEARCH. MAKE YOUR OWN CHOICES. MOVE FORWARD WHEN YOU ARE EMOTIONALLY READY AND NOT A MINUTE SOONER. ASK YOUR DOCTORS TO SLOW DOWN IF YOU FEEL THEY ARE MOVING TOO FAST. CREATE BOUNDARIES. PUSH AWAY THE PEOPLE WHO ARE OVERLY FEARFUL AND ANXIOUS. MAKE MORE ROOM FOR THOSE WHO BRING YOU PEACE AND SUPPORT.

I became my own advocate and indulged in many visits to Dr. Google

When I first met with my surgeon, he told me that he could schedule my radical surgery in two weeks. Immediately my brain said, "Slow down Cowboy!" I explained to him that for me to fully focus on healing after the surgery, I needed time to get my ducks in a row. I had some big work projects that needed to be wrapped up and I needed time to spend with my girlfriends who would be my support system while I healed. He understood and recommended a time frame that would allow me to prepare emotionally. I checked my calendar and scheduled a surgery date that worked for ME.

Doctors are human and I believe all but a very few are trying to heal their patients. But they have hundreds of patients and you are only one of many. It is not their job, nor the job of their administrative staff to lead and guide you through Cancer. They don't have time or the resources for hand holding. I mean no disrespect for the Doctors or their staff. I am aware of the financial constraints of a medical office. You must become your own advocate and find others who have gone before you on a similar journey to help you along.

Dr. Google directed me to a YouTube video of a dear woman who is tops on my list of Healing Heroes. Once my bladder was removed, they would need to send my urine someplace else. I had a few options to choose from. They could make a new bladder, hook it up to the old pipes and I would pee "normally" but most likely be incontinent during the day and certainly incontinent during the night. (Insert eye roll here) This was not a good option for me. Another option was to wear an external bag that would collect urine. Ugh! I searched Google for hours looking for someone that looked sexy while wearing a urostomy bag under their clothes. Nothing ever turned up sexy enough to satisfy me. The last option was "continent urinary diversion" (aka Indiana Pouch aka Bionic Woman option). This option removes the bladder, creates an internal reservoir (pouch) from healthy intestine allowing access to the reservoir from a stoma on the abdomen. I Googled Indiana Pouch and found a video of a lady demonstrating her process to drain her Indiana

Pouch. I was streaming tears of joy by the time she was done. I could do this! She made it look so easy. I could totally do this!

I emailed my surgeon and asked if I was a viable candidate for this type of procedure. He confirmed that I was a very good candidate. Bionic Woman, here I come!

I joined an online Bladder Cancer Advocacy Network which was incredibly valuable after my surgery but a holy terror beforehand. Online support groups are typically dominated by people who are having complications and problems. I learned quickly not to read the posts every day. I learned how to search for the answer to questions specific to me. When I needed advice, the network was supportive and made great suggestions. Someone even directed me to a blog written by a doctor with an Indiana Pouch Blog that answered every possible question I could imagine and others I never would have thought of. Thanks to the blog I keep a "Go Bag" stuffed with needed catheters and medical supplies to last for a week in case of emergency.

The surgery pathology report revealed that Cancer was microscopically evident in two of my lymph nodes. This is considered a very bad outcome. The Cancer had spread beyond my bladder. I was under the impression that the next step was chemo. The day came to meet with the Oncologist. He went over all the data and statistics with me related to Bladder Cancer and chemo. The condensed version of his info is that having chemo would only improve my odds of non-recurrence by 7% over someone who didn't go through Chemo. My friend Jackie was with me in the room and listening along with me. I thanked the Oncologist for the information and told him I'd like to take some time to think about the information he gave me before making my decision. When he walked out of the room I looked at Jackie and declared, "Oh Hell no! There is no Effin way I'm having chemo for so little a result! I'll eat more broccoli and probably get a better outcome!" I was my own advocate. I considered what was best for me and chose not to have chemo. (Insert disclaimer here!!! I do not recommend that everyone refuse chemo. It made sense in my situation, with my type of cancer and at my age. You need to ask for data and statistics, or do your own research, regarding what is best for you in your situation)

BECOME YOUR OWN ADVOCATE

BE YOUR OWN ADVOCATE. THIS IS YOUR JOURNEY. DO YOUR OWN RESEARCH. MAKE YOUR OWN CHOICES. MOVE FORWARD WHEN YOU ARE EMOTIONALLY READY AND NOT A MINUTE SOONER. ASK YOUR DOCTORS TO SLOW DOWN IF YOU FEEL THEY ARE MOVING TOO FAST. CREATE BOUNDARIES. PUSH AWAY THE PEOPLE WHO ARE OVERLY FEARFUL AND ANXIOUS. MAKE MORE ROOM FOR THOSE WHO BRING YOU PEACE AND SUPPORT.

Take a moment...write your thoughts or pause for reflection.

What are you doing to advocate for yourself? Are you getting all the information you need from your Physician? Are you getting the support you need from the people closest to you? Is there anyone who you need to back away from due to their negativity? If you were to share advice on advocacy for a friend that was diagnosed, what would you say and how would you advocate for them?

♥

CONCEPT TEN

LET GO OF EXPECTATIONS AND THE WAY THINGS HAVE ALWAYS BEEN

TAKE THE TIME TO CREATE A CEREMONY TO HONOR AND ACKNOWLEDGE THIS GREAT LIFE PASSAGE AND/OR CANCER EXPERIENCE. INVITE YOUR CLOSEST FRIENDS TO EXPERIENCE THIS WITH YOU. I HAVE A YOUNG FRIEND WHO WAS DIAGNOSED WITH BREAST CANCER WHO HAD A "SAY GOODBYE TO THE BOOBIES" PARTY BEFORE HER DOUBLE MASTECTOMY. IF THE THOUGHT OF A PARTY IS TOO UNCOMFORTABLE FOR YOU, THEN SET ASIDE AN HOUR OF PEACE, SOLITUDE AND CONTEMPLATION. LIGHT A CANDLE, POUR A SOOTHING CUP OF TEA OR GLASS OF WINE AND WRITE A LETTER OF GRATITUDE TO YOUR BODY FOR ITS YEARS OF LOYALTY AND TO THIS AMAZING JOURNEY YOU'LL CONTINUE TO SHARE TOGETHER.

It was time to say good bye to the black string bikini.

All great life passages involve a ceremony or rite of passage. We have graduations, baptisms, birthday parties, anniversaries and weddings. I felt that my surgery would be one of my greatest life passages and needed to be acknowledged, honored or celebrated in some way.

I knew that my life would be different after the surgery. But I had no point of reference for what it would be like. I only knew one thing…I would have to retire the black string bikini. My friend Nicole asked me how she could help me in my journey. I told her we needed to have a ceremony to mark this great life passage. Let's have a "say goodbye to the black sting bikini" ceremony. So, the week before my surgery, Nicole arranged an evening that included our friend Hope. The three of us enjoyed a good meal then spent an hour sipping champagne in Nicole's hot tub under a star filled winter night and I wore my black string bikini one last time.

Before you think I am extremely shallow for being concerned about being able to wear a bikini, let me clarify what was really going on…

My body was about to change. Organs would be removed; other organs would be repurposed and I would have a nifty little hole (stoma) in my abdomen that would allow me to drain body fluids on command. It would be necessary to always wear an absorbent pad over the stoma to protect this new fragile little body part. My body would be different. The "ceremony" wasn't about saying good bye to the black string bikini. It was about saying good bye to the body who had served me so well for 58 years. It was about formally marking a great life passage and saying goodbye to the past and emotionally preparing for the future.

After sitting in the jacuzzi for a while, I could feel my mood change. I wanted to be alone. I stepped out of the hot tub, wrapped myself in a towel and said good night to my friends. They wished me good luck on my surgery then I drove home in silence and solitude. Tears streamed down my face as I mentally thanked my body for the years of dependable service it had already provided. I acknowledged the transformation that we would endure in the coming months. I gave honor to the significance of this amazing adventure and life altering experience my body and I were sharing. I went to bed that night, a little sad and felt warm tears slowly fill my eyes again and roll down my cheeks.

The next morning, ceremony now over, I was emotionally ready to move forward.

LET GO OF EXPECTATIONS AND THE WAY THINGS HAVE ALWAYS BEEN

TAKE THE TIME TO CREATE A CEREMONY TO HONOR AND ACKNOWLEDGE THIS GREAT LIFE PASSAGE AND/OR CANCER EXPERIENCE. INVITE YOUR CLOSEST FRIENDS TO EXPERIENCE THIS WITH YOU. I HAVE A YOUNG FRIEND WHO WAS DIAGNOSED WITH BREAST CANCER WHO HAD A "SAY GOODBYE TO THE BOOBIES" PARTY BEFORE HER DOUBLE MASTECTOMY. IF THE THOUGHT OF A PARTY IS TOO UNCOMFORTABLE FOR YOU, THEN SET ASIDE AN HOUR OF PEACE, SOLITUDE AND CONTEMPLATION. LIGHT A CANDLE, POUR A SOOTHING CUP OF TEA OR GLASS OF WINE AND WRITE A LETTER OF GRATITUDE TO YOUR BODY FOR ITS YEARS OF LOYALTY AND TO THIS AMAZING JOURNEY YOU'LL CONTINUE TO SHARE TOGETHER.

Take a moment...write your thoughts or pause for reflection.

Create a ceremony, rite of passage or celebration to honor this significant time in your life.

CONCEPT ELEVEN

PREPARE LIKE YOU'RE GOING ON VACATION

BUY NEW CLOTHES, GET YOUR HAIR DONE, GET A MANICURE, CLEAN THE FRIDGE, UPDATE YOUR WILL AND SHOW SOMEONE WHERE YOU KEEP YOUR PASSWORDS. RELIEVE YOURSELF OF THE STRESS OF THE DAILY GRIND SO THAT YOU CAN FULLY FOCUS ON HEALING.

There wasn't a manual to prepare for radical Cancer surgery. So, I decided to prepare for a vacation instead. Everything needed to be handled before I checked into the hospital. I wanted to be able to focus on healing and nothing else. I already mentioned that my surgeon was prepared to schedule me pronto. But I needed time to prepare. The biggest tasks were related to work projects I wanted to complete so I could "let go" of work responsibility. I had the projects wrapped up several days early. I made an extensive list of major and minor tasks that I needed to accomplish before I could fully embrace and appreciate a long hospital stay. I desired to have the freedom to relax and heal completely stress free.

I took on some "minor" household projects that I knew would make things easier for me when I returned home from the hospital. I cleaned out closets and drawers and sent several bags of old clothes to charity. I stocked up on home essentials like napkins, paper plates and Styrofoam cups. I cleaned out the fridge of leftovers and food we were never going to consume. I wiped the shelves and the racks so that they sparkled. I contacted a cleaning lady and asked her to do a major spring cleaning of my house. The kitchen, bathroom, mirrors, windows and shutters looked like I was ready to entertain guests.

My pre-op appointment provided me with some essential information on what to expect after surgery. I was aware that I would return home with multiple tubes coming from my abdomen and a fluid collection bag to strap to my leg. My week-long encounter with a catheter and collection bag after the outpatient procedure was all the education I needed to be better prepared this time. I purchased several elastic waist full length skirts that would make it easy to access all the equipment underneath while also covering up all the tubes, tape and bag. The skirts I bought were lovely and contributed to a beautiful state of mind that helped with my recovery. I may have been sick, but I didn't have to look the part.

I paid all my bills and utilities for two months. I pulled all my financial information together (Life Insurance, Health Insurance, banking, charge cards, and investments) so that it would be easy for someone else to find if necessary. I made sure my Will/Living Trust was current and added a note inside the binder regarding my intentions and wishes on how my son might budget an inheritance (Do Not buy a new car!!!). I reminded my cousin Ed that he was the Trustee and gave him a copy of the Will/Living Trust. I taped a big note to the drawer that held all these valuable papers so that, if the worst happened, my son would know where to find his next step.

I set an "out of office notification" on my email with phone numbers of other business partners who could assist my clients during my absence. I changed the voicemail message on my phone to provide alternative phone numbers for more assistance. I'm a business owner and work independently. I'd heard of other Health Insurance Agents who passed away unexpectedly and their family members lost the business income due to a lack of knowledge and/or contingency plan. So, I called Jonathan, a fellow Agent who I trust and respect, and let him know that if the worst happened I needed him to take over my business and share the commissions with my son. I taped a big note to my computer with Jonathan's contact info and instructions. Both my son and Jonathan had a copy. Jonathan had access to all my work-related passwords and I trusted my son with my personal password book and debit card.

I made appointments to get my hair done (trimmed and highlighted) and had my nails done. Beauty, or at least feeling beautiful, is more important when you're sick especially if you know you are going to be out of commission recovering for long periods. During my recovery, it became very important to me to look like myself and less like a patient. So, get your hair and nails done before things get rough.

I wrote out daily instructions to my son on household chores to handle while I was gone. *Feed the dog, water the potted plants, check the mail, be sure the doors are locked before you go to work, don't run the air conditioner while you're away from home.*

The day before my hospital stay, I laundered my bedding and changed my sheets. I love getting into a clean bed with fresh sheets and I knew that I would appreciate it more than ever before after being in a hospital bed. I packed a small bag with a change of clothes to wear home from the hospital. I added several hours of my favorite podcasts to my iPod and made a peaceful healing music playlist. I also packed a household extension cord and charging cables so that I could easily keep my phone and iPod powered up and easily accessible while stuck in a hospital bed.

There were things I should have prepared for differently. I wish I would have cleared ALL the clutter and decorations from my bedroom side tables before I went to the hospital. I needed space for all the post-op stuff that is critical after surgery. Before I went into the hospital, I should have purchased a medical shower chair. My son had to scramble to purchase a walker and shower chair before the hospital would release me.

Let the trivial things slide. Don't sweat the small stuff. I knew that my son probably wouldn't clean the kitchen to my satisfaction so I stayed out. I threw a sheet over my easy chair and love seat so that I didn't have to worry about staining or soiling the fabric. Everywhere I went in the house I laid down towels under my fluid collection bag. It wasn't pretty, but I didn't have to worry about leaking and ruining my furniture or carpeting.

Preparing and organizing your life as if you are going on vacation makes it easy to focus on healing. In my case, I was preparing for a long hospital stay and radical surgery. But you might be starting with chemo. I encourage you to prepare for a different lifestyle before the chemo starts.

PREPARE LIKE YOU'RE GOING ON VACATION

BUY NEW CLOTHES, GET YOUR HAIR DONE, GET A MANICURE, CLEAN THE FRIDGE, UPDATE YOUR WILL AND SHOW SOMEONE WHERE YOU KEEP YOUR PASSWORDS. RELIEVE YOURSELF OF THE STRESS OF THE DAILY GRIND SO THAT YOU CAN FULLY FOCUS ON HEALING.

Take a moment...write your thoughts or pause for reflection.

What do you need to do to prepare now so that things will be easier for you later? Make a list...a long list. Are there things you can delegate to someone else?

CONCEPT TWELVE

ALLOW YOURSELF THE SPACE TO HEAL.

CREATE A HEALING ENVIRONMENT WITH POSITIVE MESSAGES, SOOTHING MUSIC AND LOVELY FRAGRANCE. FIND YOUR HAPPY PLACE AND SPEND TIME THERE OFTEN. SURROUND YOURSELF WITH HEALING VISUAL IMAGES AND PROGRAM YOUR SUBCONSCIOUS FOR A POSITIVE EXPERIENCE.

YOU MUST GIVE YOURSELF PERMISSION TO FOCUS AND PRIORITIZE HEALING. THIS MEANS CREATING AN ENVIRONMENT TO HEAL EVEN IF IT MEANS CREATING BOUNDARIES TO KEEP NEGATIVE PEOPLE AND THINKING OUT.

As soon as I was diagnosed with Cancer, I was focused and determine to do everything in my power to create a peaceful healing space and become Cancer free. I'm a big believer in the power of the subconscious as the lens and/or filter from which we view the world. Example: If you fill your mind with hours of Network News, you're going to program your mind to see the world only as a place of tragedy, crime, war, pestilence and severe weather. Your Cancer experience will mimic the tragedy and drama of the evening news. You will be filled with fear and the anxiety that accompanies watching one tragedy after another. But if you fill your mind with messages of hope, peace and healing then your Cancer experience will mimic those feelings.

I love my cozy little house. Shortly after my Cancer diagnosis I made more of an effort to keep my house tidy. My office is in my home which provides me with the good fortune of being able to regulate my work environment. I made a point to light scented candles each day. I played smooth jazz and spa music to help me remain calm. I printed healing messages in big bold letters and taped them in my office and throughout the house. I AM CREATED TO LIVE A LONG HEALTHY LIFE and MY BODY IS FILLED WITH HEALING ENERGY. I didn't have to read these messages every day to allow them to seep into my subconscious. I simply needed to be exposed to them multiple times during the day to adopt them into my thought pattern. In addition, I've mentioned before, I have decorative graphic wall art throughout my house that has completely saturated my brain. A large wooden graphic of Louis Armstrong's Wonderful World dominates the wall you see as soon as you enter my house, *I see trees of green, red roses too, I see them bloom for me and you, and I think to myself, what a wonderful world.* God, I love that song. In my living room above the TV screen hangs a wooden plaque with the line from a famous Christmas movie. The plaque reads "It's A Wonderful Life." I keep this plaque up all year round.

Now that my bladder cancer surgery is over and I am the proud owner of a bionic body, my routine to drain the urine from my body requires the use of a long rubber catheter 4 -5 times a day. To insert the catheter into my stoma I need to relax and slightly recline. I intentionally installed another plaque that reads "It's a Wonderful Life" in the exact spot that my eyes move to when I am reclining and feeding a catheter into my stoma. The message just keeps imprinting its positivity into my subconscious. Instead of my draining process being emotionally painful and burdensome, it is often the most peaceful part of my day focusing on the wonder of life and how fortunate I am.

I'm an introvert and thrive in my little cozy house. It's my happy place. My adult son (age 23) was still living at home with me when I was diagnosed. I quickly began to embrace Cancer as a wonderful adventure filled with amazing life lessons. I was beginning each day dedicating five minutes to Cancer and then letting it go. But my poor son was processing the experience in complete contrast to me. He would come home after work filled with tension and anxiety. You could see it in his body language and hear the anger in his voice. He became short tempered and hostile. It was like he was dripping negative energy and splashing fear and anxiety all over my happy cozy healing space every time he walked in the door.   One evening, when he returned home from work, I invited him to take a seat in the easy chair. It was time for a heart to heart talk. I explained to him that my home was going to be my healing place for the next several months and I needed him to treat it like it was sacred space. No hostility, negativity, fear or anxiety was welcomed in my home. He would need to find a way to let go of those emotions before he came home from work each day. I told him that my healing was so important to me, if he couldn't get his emotions under control, I would have to ask him to move out. Suddenly his tense angry shoulders fell. Tears filled his eyes and his fear finally worked its way to the surface. He cried, "But you're my mom, what if you…" He was so emotional, he couldn't speak. I finished the sentence for him. "What if I die? Well, so be it. I will have lived a wonderful happy life. I have been the most fortunate woman in the world. But, Sweetheart, I'm not going to die from Cancer. I'm sure of it. I'm going to keep going and live a long and healthy life." Later I discovered, after our heart to heart talk, that my son began parking his truck in front of the neighborhood park each evening for several minutes before he returned home. He would use the time to tone down his emotions before entering my sacred healing space.

ALLOW YOURSELF THE SPACE TO HEAL. CREATE A HEALING ENVIRONMENT WITH POSITIVE MESSAGES, SOOTHING MUSIC AND LOVELY FRAGRANCE. FIND YOUR HAPPY PLACE AND SPEND TIME THERE OFTEN. SURROUND YOURSELF WITH HEALING VISUAL IMAGES AND PROGRAM YOUR SUBCONSCIOUS FOR A POSITIVE EXPERIENCE.

YOU MUST GIVE YOURSELF PERMISSION TO FOCUS AND PRIORITIZE HEALING. THIS MEANS CREATING AN ENVIRONMENT TO HEAL EVEN IF IT MEANS CREATING BOUNDARIES TO KEEP NEGATIVE PEOPLE AND THINKING OUT.

Take a moment...write your thoughts or pause for reflection.

What will you do to create a more peaceful healing space for yourself?

♥

CONCEPT THIRTEEN

LEARN TO RECEIVE

LEARN TO RECEIVE GRACIOUSLY. LET GO OF BEING IN CONTROL, IN CHARGE AND PERFECT. EMBRACE YOUR EMOTIONAL AND PHYSICAL VULNERABILITY. SAY "YES" WHEN PEOPLE OFFER TO HELP. TELL THEM THEIR EFFORT MEANS THE WORLD TO YOU. REALIZE THAT OTHERS WANT TO CONTRIBUTE AND PARTICIPATE IN YOUR RECOVERY AND SHARE YOUR JOURNEY. ALLOW THEM THE GIFT AND PRIVILEGE OF PARTICIPATING THROUGH GIVING.

I grew up in church being taught that it was better to give than receive. We gave to the poor, the needy, the sick, the helpless, the hungry, the old and the dependent. As givers, we positioned our status as being "better off", stronger, stable, responsible and independent. In my church, it wasn't respectable to be on the receiving end.

As an adult, I was uncomfortable with receiving. There is something about receiving that made me feel awkward, dependent and vulnerable. I'm a much better giver than I am a receiver.

The dynamic between myself and my brother and sister changed during Cancer. Both called me far more often than usual. We have always led very independent lives from each other. But one of us getting Cancer while we were all still so young, active and healthy wasn't something any of us ever anticipated. I think it made us all feel vulnerable. I appreciated their phone calls more than all the others. It isn't what we said or what we talked about that made the difference. It was their simple effort of reaching out that kept me from feeling as if I was in this alone. Their calls told me they were with me on this journey.

Receiving requires vulnerability. Letting my community know I had Cancer was a very difficult decision for me. It meant letting people know that I wasn't perfect, I had weakness and I wasn't in control. Receiving the love, care, sympathy and kind words of my community was uncomfortable. It was appreciated, but still uncomfortable. So, one of my beautiful lessons of Cancer was to learn to receive and do it graciously.

I was a reluctant receiver. The original plan was a short outpatient surgery to remove the bladder tumor and I would be home by lunch time and take a little Tylenol. I just needed a ride to and from the hospital. My son took the day off work to be my driver. Things didn't go as planned to say the least. I was sent home on heavy pain killers wearing a catheter attached to a fluid collection bag. I slept all day and through the night except for the two times my son stood me up (still heavily medicated) next to the bed, laid down plastic and towels on the floor in front of me, covered his hands with two layers of latex gloves and proceeded to remove a bag filled with oddly colored bodily fluid and chemo solution. I remember looking down at him and saying, "I don't recall this part being in the Cancer Adventure brochure." I was so amazed and appreciative of my son's willingness to be a Giver that day. I didn't find out until much later that the hospital wouldn't release me unless he agreed to be trained on how to empty and change the collection bag and handle the chemo solution. My reluctance of receiving changed. I realized that there would be many parts of this experience I couldn't handle alone.

Sam continued to step up to the plate to help whenever I needed and I was better at surrendering and letting him take over. After the second surgery, I was pretty darn helpless. I needed help getting in and out of bed and navigating around a yard of tubes and two fluid collection bags. Nightly, I'd get situated in bed and Sam would make sure the tubes and bags were positioned without kinks. He insisted we sleep with our bedroom doors open so he could hear me in the middle of the night if I needed help. I felt loved.

My most precious moment of receiving was the week after my second surgery. My son drove me back to the Cancer Center to check in with the doctor. Sam dropped me off in front of the hospital while he parked the car. I sat on a bench in the San Diego sun, weak and exhausted holding a grocery bag that contained my two fluid collection bags. I sat and watched while sick people passed by. They dragged oxygen tanks, hid their bald heads with scarves, shuffled slowly by pushing walkers and sat hunched over while being pushed in wheel chairs. To me, they looked like they were on their last days and I wondered which ones would survive. It scared me. I realized I was one of them. I felt weak and scared and wanted to weep but I held it in. My son held my arm as I slowly made my way into the hospital reception area. I went to the restroom to drain my urine bag when I finally started crying. Tears just kept rolling down my cheeks. I felt feeble, helpless and frightened. I splashed cold water on my face hoping Sam wouldn't know I was crying. But as soon as I stepped into the hall he took one look at me and knew. Sam put his big strong arm around sick little me and I buried my face in his great big chest and cried. He kissed the top of my head and told me it would be okay. What a precious moment it was to receive the love and support of my great big boy. It was a new beautiful shift in our mother/son relationship.

Receiving graciously is the difference between saying to the friend who brings a casserole, "Oh no, you shouldn't have gone to the trouble", but instead learning to say "Thank you for bringing a casserole. It means so much to me that you made the effort."

People offered to help in any way I needed and I had to learn to let them. "Yes, I need a ride to the Doctor and its 2 hours away in traffic. Yes, I would love it if you brought food. Yes, I need someone to come sort through all my medical supplies. Yes, please come with me when I speak to the Oncologist about chemo. Yes, please come with me when the doctor teaches me how to use the catheter." And to my sister, "Yes, it meant the world to me that you were there for me from the first moment I was diagnosed and came to the hospital every day. I will never forget. It meant the world to me."

Receiving was difficult at first but became easier and I felt more comfortable allowing friends to help. I began to let go of my need to be in control, in charge and independent. I realized that my Cancer experience was a journey that was intended to be shared and important to those who participated with me.

LEARN TO RECEIVE GRACIOUSLY. LET GO OF BEING IN CONTROL, IN CHARGE AND PERFECT. EMBRACE YOUR EMOTIONAL AND PHYSICAL VULNERABILITY. SAY "YES" WHEN PEOPLE OFFER TO HELP. TELL THEM THEIR EFFORT MEANS THE WORLD TO YOU. REALIZE THAT OTHERS WANT TO CONTRIBUTE AND PARTICIPATE IN YOUR RECOVERY AND SHARE YOUR JOURNEY. ALLOW THEM THE GIFT AND PRIVILEGE OF PARTICIPATING THROUGH GIVING.

Take a moment...write your thoughts or pause for reflection.

If you haven't already, find a way to thank the people who have helped you and supported you on this Journey. Are you uncomfortable with receiving? Prepare yourself to say "yes" to the next person who offers to help.

CONCEPT FOURTEEN

FIND A SUPPORT GROUP

FIND A SUPPORT GROUP RELATED TO YOUR SPECIFIC CANCER. ACCLIMATE SLOWLY AND EASE INTO IT LIKE YOU'RE STEPPING INTO CHILLY WATER. ADJUST SLOWLY AND WHEN NECESSARY EASE BACK WHEN THE INFORMATION FEELS FRIGHTENING AND OVERWHELMING. REMEMBER THAT EVENTUALLY THE TIME WILL COME TO LET GO OF YOUR SUPPORT GROUP AND THRIVE.

Find a support group specific to your type of cancer. It can be a face to face support group or it can be an online support group. But ease in slowly like walking into chilly water. Acclimate slowly.

I stumbled across Bladder Cancer Advocacy Network through a Google search. It's an online support group specific to people with Bladder Cancer. I created a basic profile so that I could search the network and read the posts and responses. I would log in a couple of times a day to see the latest trending posts. But truthfully, it was frightening. I was still very healthy in the beginning. But every time I logged into the network I would see posts from patients who were struggling with everything and anything related to Cancer that could possibly go wrong. Chemo, nausea, surgery, abscesses, infections, leaking urostomy pouches, catheters, repeated surgeries, bad doctors, bad hospitals and an unlimited number of abbreviations for common bladder related terminology (none of which I understood). Every post I read by the support group caused heavy amounts of anxiety for me. There weren't any "super successful bladder cancer stories" popping up. And that's what I expected from a support platform. So, I drastically cut back on my virtual visits to the network in hopes of maintaining a positive outlook and optimistic frame of mind.

In Concept Six, Words Have Power, I shared how I revealed my diagnosis with friends and acquaintances on Facebook. Letting my community know that I had been diagnosed resulted in mountains of support. *A problem shared is a problem halved.* By sharing my "problem" I reduced the weight of the burden I was carrying.

As my Cancer journey progressed, I needed the help of people who had already walked in my shoes and it was time to return to the Bladder Cancer Advocacy Network. But instead of reading random posts I would run searches for answers to my specific question. If I couldn't find what I needed, I would create an original post and I always received useful information from other Bladder Cancer patients. My specific procedure / solution is referred to as an Indiana Pouch (IP is the recognized abbreviation in Bladder Cancer Land). I was comfortable spending more time on the Network but would limit my reading only to posts of other IP patients. It resulted in my ability to be proactive in my healing after my surgery. Eventually, I found the one post I wanted to read more than any other. Another IP patient posted "Life with IP is better than normal. If you have an IP, post a photo of you doing something amazing." What followed were photos of Indiana Pouch patients skiing, scuba diving, back packing and sky diving. Not only did I feel supported, I felt inspired and motivated and looked forward to riding my bike again.

I used to check in sporadically to the Bladder Cancer Advocacy Network and run a search for the latest posts by other Indiana Pouch patients. My prognosis and recovery has been ideal and text book perfect. But I am reminded that support groups are typically made up of people who need support and are struggling with their health and recovery. Many people with an Indiana Pouch post about urine leakage and random squirting. The last post I read was related to a woman who has had her Indiana Pouch for more than five years. She was seeking support and advice because her stoma unpredictably leaks large amounts of urine and she fears leaving her house. I could feel my body switch to hyper anxiety mode fearing that it could happen to me in the future. I decided to stop participating on the Bladder Cancer Advocacy Network because it was scaring the crap out of me.

Eventually, it's time to let go of your support group and learn to thrive. But if you're familiar with any recovery program, whether it is addiction or disease, the last step is about sharing your recovery with others to help someone else in their healing process. In my career as a Health Insurance Agent, I have the pleasure of talking to people newly diagnosed with Cancer. With compassion and understanding, I assist them with their Health Insurance and coach them to find peace during a challenging time. Maybe I will return to the Bladder Cancer Advocacy Network as a survivor in the future when the experience is more historical and not as current as it is today.

FIND A SUPPORT GROUP RELATED TO YOUR SPECIFIC CANCER. ACCLIMATE SLOWLY AND EASE INTO IT LIKE YOU'RE STEPPING INTO CHILLY WATER. ADJUST SLOWLY AND WHEN NECESSARY EASE BACK WHEN THE INFORMATION FEELS FRIGHTENING AND OVERWHELMING. REMEMBER THAT EVENTUALLY THE TIME WILL COME TO LET GO OF YOUR SUPPORT GROUP AND THRIVE.

Take a moment...write your thoughts or pause for reflection.

If you haven't already, find a support group specific to your type of Cancer. It can be an online group or one that meets face to face on a consistent basis. You can Google the type of Cancer you have and add the words "support group near me". If necessary, find a Grief Counselor to help you through this process.

♥

CONCEPT FIFTEEN

FLIP THE RESET SWITCH

CANCER CAN PROVIDE A FABULOUS RESET SWITCH THAT ALLOWS A PERSON TO CREATE AND CHOOSE A NEW MORE INTENTIONAL LIFE. THE RESET SWITCH MIGHT NUDGE THEM INTO SKYDIVING AND MARATHON RUNNING OR HEALTHY EATING, YOGA AND MEDITATION. CANCER GIVES THE MARVELOUS GIFT OF THE RESET SWITCH.

My Cancer, although invasive and potentially life threatening, didn't have any significant impact on my daily life or activities prior to my surgery. I felt fine. I felt normal. I felt healthy. I was full of energy. My life was active and busy. I ran my own business and attended several networking events and social gatherings each month. I met girlfriends for lunch, dinner and happy hour. Life was full and fabulous.

Then came the surgery. After only a week in the hospital I returned home. I had tubes coming out of everywhere. One of the tubes had to remain attached for 2 months. I truly hated that tube. It was horribly uncomfortable and painful. It limited my movements and worst of all altered my frame of mind. When you're in constant pain, even if it's mild pain, it becomes difficult to concentrate. Still recovering from surgery, I found myself exhausted most of the time. I didn't want to do anything other than try to find a comfortable position that would reduce the pain and catch another nap.

My life was made up of multiple daily catnaps. Rarely did I stay awake for more than a couple of hours. I didn't even have the energy to watch a new movie. Trying to focus or concentrate on a movie plot was of no interest to me so I watched Downton Abby reruns. I love to read, but found it difficult to focus on the pages of a book or the screen on my Kindle. Friends would call to check in on me but I really didn't like giving health updates all day long. I didn't have the energy to say, "I'm tired, I hurt and I hate this stupid tube!" so I let the calls go to voice mail instead.

So, there I was for two months…doing nothing more than napping and healing. If nothing else, I was PRESENT. I couldn't make plans for my future or set exciting business goals because I didn't know if the Cancer was gone or if I would have to go through Chemotherapy. I took life hour by hour. Nap to nap. *It was awesome.* I'm not kidding!

Imagine having no expectations of yourself. Imagine getting to hit a reset switch on your entire life. All the stuff that clutters your life is temporarily washed away. Your schedule is cleared. No one expects you to answer the phone, clean the house, go shopping, run a business, show up to social events, participate in business networking, put on makeup, stay up on current events, exercise, cook or even drive a car.

Cancer had gifted me a giant RESET SWITCH. What a treat! When my health returned, I could build my life intentionally instead of accidently. I could be strategic about how to spend my time, energy and effort. I could operate my life from a new fresh perspective. As soon as the last tube was removed, I started to create my life.

How I spent my time and who I spent my time with changed. I said "NO" much more often. I was more selective with accepting invitations. I dressed for comfort rather than dressing to impress. The first thing to eliminate was the desire for the bikini bod. My motivation for healthy eating shifted from trying to impress others with a slim physique to making sure my new body parts would work well.

All those networking events I used to attend were now a chore in which I found very little joy or benefit. I realized they had become a habit and routine that I had never taken the time to evaluate. So, I decided to limit my networking to just a few events that held great benefit for me personally and say NO to the rest. This freed up my time and energy considerably.

Parties and social gatherings were whittled down significantly too. My new body parts require inconvenient maintenance every few hours. I don't let it limit my life in any way. But the inconvenience is just enough to make the timing of my social outings intentional. I'd much rather handle the bionic body maintenance at home. I attend fewer but richer activities than I did before.

I have always felt like I should maintain a connection to every person in my past regardless if we still had anything in common. No longer. Now that my slate was wiped clean and the reset switch was triggered, I became intentional with my "friend energy". Today, when I think of old friends with whom I have lost close contact, I mentally send them a virtual hug, wish them well and feel grateful that we had shared a portion of the journey together. And then I let go unless our paths conveniently cross again.

Quiet time is more important to me than ever before. I don't know that I ever gave quiet time any priority before my surgery. Life was full and fast back then. Slow and steady works better for me now and I choose to stop and smell the roses more often. Today I enjoy feelings of constant peace and calm where before life was a constant barrage of energy and activity. Embrace the reset switch and create an intentional life.

CANCER CAN PROVIDE A FABULOUS RESET SWITCH THAT ALLOWS A PERSON TO CREATE AND CHOOSE A NEW MORE INTENTIONAL LIFE. THE RESET SWITCH MIGHT NUDGE THEM INTO SKYDIVING AND MARATHON RUNNING OR HEALTHY EATING, YOGA AND MEDITATION. CANCER GIVES THE MARVELOUS GIFT OF THE RESET SWITCH.

Take a moment...write your thoughts or pause for reflection.

When this is over and it's time to create a new normal, what would you like to eliminate from your life and what would you like to add?

♥

CONCEPT SIXTEEN

CHOOSE HUMOR OVER HUMILIATION

THERE'S NOTHING FUNNY ABOUT CANCER.

WAIT! OH, YES THERE IS!

WHEN GIVEN THE CHOICE BETWEEN HUMILIATION AND HUMOR, CHOOSE HUMOR.

DURING A CANCER JOURNEY, THERE WILL BE MANY OPPORTUNITIES IN WHICH YOU WILL HAVE TO MAKE A CHOICE BETWEEN HUMILIATION OR HUMOR. STUDIES HAVE ALREADY PROVEN THE BENEFITS OF LAUGHTER FOR THE HEALING PROCESS. LAUGHTER MAKES YOU FEEL BETTER EMOTIONALLY. SCIENTIFIC STUDIES REVEAL IT REDUCES PAIN, IMPROVES YOUR IMMUNE SYSTEM AND AIDS IN BRAIN FUNCTION. SO, FIND THE HUMOR IN EACH SITUATION AND LAUGH YOUR ASS OFF WHENEVER YOU CAN!

I lost track of all the weird and wild moments in my journey that caused me to shake my head and laugh at the lunacy of the situation. I could have cried, but laughing produced better results and made my Cancer adventure bearable.

I didn't have all the necessary medical supplies I required when I first came home from the hospital. I needed a large irrigation syringe to keep the tubes attached to the urine bags clear. My sister went to every pharmacy and Medical Supply store in the valley but to no avail. Eventually she returned home with a turkey baster. It was the craziest most perfect solution ever! I will spare you the crazy gross details of our first attempt using the turkey baster. But, it worked great, almost too great, and I giggle every time I think of it!

My friend Adria went with me the day my surgeon taught me how to "self-cath" (insert a catheter into my abdominal stoma to drain urine from my internal reservoir). This was a big emotional step in my healing and the rest of my life. I was nervous and kind of grossed out by the process. I was grateful to have a supportive friend with me. On our way home, Adria cracked me up when she pointed out that the Doctor's instruction on the cathing process sounded a lot like instructions on sex. "First, generously cover with lubricant then insert slowly. It might be tight, so relax. If there is resistance, back it out a little and try again. Add more lubricant if needed. It should slide in and out easily." We laughed all the way home.

The best example of choosing humor over humiliation was my very first attempt at self-cathing at home. I needed to measure my output so I drained into a plastic measuring container. Everything went well and I felt very proud of my first attempt. That is, until the container of urine slipped out of my hand, hit the floor and splashed all over me and the bathroom. While standing covered in urine, there was a split second of shock in which my emotions could have swung in either direction. I could have cried and wallowed in self-pity that this was an indicator of what would be the path for the rest of my life. But I chose to laugh in the moment, cleaned up the mess and forge a path that would set a positive trajectory for the rest of my life realizing I would need to keep a stronger grip on all future containers of urine.

There have been an unlimited number of, what could have been, awkward humiliating moments during my healing process. But sprinkled with a dose of humor, those moments have become great lessons in my Cancer journey.

(Side note, there were also times when I wallowed in brief little pity parties when I just didn't have the strength or stamina to choose humor. Laugh when you can, but when you can't, let the tears roll. Don't hold back.)

WHEN GIVEN THE CHOICE BETWEEN HUMILIATION AND HUMOR, CHOOSE HUMOR.

DURING A CANCER JOURNEY, THERE WILL BE MANY OPPORTUNITIES IN WHICH YOU WILL HAVE TO MAKE A CHOICE BETWEEN HUMILIATION OR HUMOR. STUDIES HAVE ALREADY PROVEN THE BENEFITS OF LAUGHTER FOR THE HEALING PROCESS. LAUGHTER MAKES YOU FEEL BETTER EMOTIONALLY. SCIENTIFIC STUDIES REVEAL IT REDUCES PAIN, IMPROVES YOUR IMMUNE SYSTEM AND AIDS IN BRAIN FUNCTION. SO, FIND THE HUMOR IN EACH SITUATION AND LAUGH YOUR ASS OFF WHENEVER YOU CAN!

Take a moment...write your thoughts or pause for reflection.

Have there been any weird, awkward or humiliating situations on this journey? Are you carrying the embarrassment of the situation with you? Take a moment to re-frame these situations into humor instead of humiliation.

CONCEPT SEVENTEEN

CREATE A RESPONSE TO THE QUESTION "WHAT IF?"

"I'M NOT AFRAID. I WILL EMBRACE CANCER WITH EVEN MORE INTENTION AND LESS FEAR THAN BEFORE."

There is no such thing as moving on after Cancer. Because every twinge, every ache, every pain makes you think to yourself "What if it's back." There may never come a time when you are completely able to release the vulnerability that it could happen again. Although I am Cancer free today, my Cancer journey isn't over. I am very aware that I could be diagnosed again in the future and the next experience could be very different than the first time around. So, I celebrate when I can.

The first grand anniversary is the One Year Cancer Free Anniversary. Celebrate the heck out of this giant milestone. I spent my One Year Anniversary and my 60th birthday at the foot of the Eiffel Tower in Paris, France. Prior to my diagnosis, I had no desire to travel or see the world. But "what if it comes back" is always playing on a constant loop in my subconscious and I feel compelled to do more and see more before it does. I push myself out of my comfort zone, pack my medical kit full of catheters and head out for adventure.

But, what if it comes back? Each day that passes lowers the risk of recurrence. The first two years after treatment are the most important. At five years you are even less likely to get a recurrence and after ten years a doctor might even be willing to declare "you're cured."

But while your mind might drift to worry and fear the next time you have a simple side ache, straight to the thought, "What if this is it? What if it's back?" It's good to have an answer prepared.

"What if it comes back?" a little voice in my head asks much too frequently. I answer audibly and with firm conviction "Then Cancer is wasting it's time. I'm not afraid. I will embrace it again. I will suck the marrow from the experience with even more intention and less fear than before."

PREPARE A RESPONSE TO THE "WHAT IF IT COMES BACK?" QUESTION.

"I'M NOT AFRAID. I WLL EMBRACE CANCER WITH EVEN MORE INTENTION AND LESS FEAR THAN BEFORE."

Take a moment...write your thoughts or pause for reflection.

If you are a Cancer Survivor, take some time to create a short sentence on how you will respond to Cancer again in the future if it returns.

♥

WAITING ON CANCER

I never understood what it meant to live in the present moment until I was diagnosed with Cancer. The time frame from the day I was diagnosed until I had a "clean bill of health" and could return to my normal life (new normal) was almost 7 months. During those months, I was forced to live in the present because there was no guarantee of the future.

January is one of my favorite months. I get to make resolutions, new goals, plan new life strategies, envision the future, swear to lose 10 pounds (again), create a business growth plan, plan home improvements and make vacation reservations. But I couldn't create any of those plans or strategies while addressing Cancer. I could only stay in my present experience. My future was uncertain. It was a weird feeling, like a fish out of water. By nature, I'm a future thinker. I love having something wonderful to look forward to. But in this situation, all I could do was show up each day to be present and wait on Cancer.

Now that I have established my new normal, I often feel like I am getting too far ahead of myself, too attached to my calendar and too focused on the future instead of focusing on the wonderful day at hand. I try to mentally return to my days of waiting on Cancer. I remember to be present and show up just for today and block out my excitement, anticipation and enthusiasm for the future. Each day is filled with wonder, power and peace. But to appreciate the wonder of each day and experience it fully, I must be present and give time, honor and space to TODAY.

September 26, 2017, the day I launch this book. I met with my Urologist yesterday for my six-month checkup. I am 18 months cancer free! Yay me!

FROM THE AUTHOR

I hope this book will provide you some comfort in your journey. I knew when I was diagnosed that it was up to me to determine what my Cancer experience would be like. We all have choices. I chose to have a Beautiful Cancer experience. Best wishes in your healing and lifelong quest to thrive.

ABOUT THE AUTHOR

Jami Buchanan McNees is a highly successful Health Insurance Agent. Her goal is to provide Health Insurance that will provide a financial safety net in the event of a catastrophic diagnosis. She recognizes that early detection is the key to Cancer survival and encourages her clients to create familiarity and relationship with trusted Doctors. Her Cancer experience wasn't just a journey toward healing but also an opportunity to become an expert in Health Insurance as the patient. Her career gives her the privilege to support people with a new Cancer diagnosis and desperate for answers related to Health Insurance. To contact Jami, you can email her at Jami@TheHealthInsuranceLady.com You can also get more insight and information on her Facebook page https://www.facebook.com/BeautifulCancerStories/

Made in the
USA
Lexington, KY